Preface

This book serves as a referenceable guide. As a reminder, if you or anyone you know is suffering from domestic abuse, please help them notify the proper channels available in your area to receive help.

Part 1

Presumably everyone alive today has come across a person who has the narcissistic personality disorder. Either this person was a friend, coworker, or lover. The narcissist in your life could even be you. Regardless, you will think of them without trying while you read this narrative.

A narcissistic person is smart. Not in a well-rounded sense where intellectual, emotional, and academic categories overlap. They are usually intricate thinkers with a knack for manipulation. Their entire true identity is engulfed and surrounded by a master puppet. This façade, masked masquerader, whom they use to entice, charm and lie to everyone they meet, eventually becomes the same demon that controls who they really are inside.

This exchange of power from where they are pulling the strings of their creation, to when the creation holds the cards against them, occurs as distinctly as the seasons change. No one can say the exact day and time the seasons change from one to the next. We may see snow and ice melting, uncovering bare earth for the first time in months. We witness the temperatures fighting to warm and become steady. Then suddenly it is no longer winter and spring is in full bloom. The exchange of power within a troubled individual wearing a mask happens just the same. Often times they themselves don't even realize it. Those who become partly aware are left to choose whether to give up this façade and go back to being themselves or to allow this alter ego to gain complete control. Rarely does a narcissist find the courage to be their authentic selves. Doing so means going back to honesty. The problem most times with choosing honesty is that most of the time the creator of this alter ego is fragile. They are easily affected by the slightest bit of criticism, which wounds them deeply. So, to admit they are lying or are ever wrong is something they just can't fathom the pain of doing.

They are also compulsive liars. If one day your average narcissist decided to choose honesty over the layers and layers of lies they used to create their self-perceived position of power, it would mean admitting the years and years of countless lies they have been telling everyone they ever met. Once the truth would be revealed, they would lose their followers and the endless praise from their unyielding fan club. Their fans relentlessly believe anything the narcissists says, cheers them on, and backs them up without even checking to see if what they say is true.

Their image is something they worked hard to achieve. The thought of those people learning the truth would crush the narcissists image and they would lose their following. They certainly wouldn't want to tarnish their image with the truth. So, they do what they do best. Lie. If anyone they use ever becomes wise to their scheming and leaves the relationship they had, whether friendship or romantic, the narcissist will turn on them without hesitation and spread the nastiest rumors you could ever imagine. This has been referenced as the grand smear campaign. Above all the things they will want you to believe, is that this person is mentally unstable. If they can get as many strangers to turn against someone they never met and believe this person is mentally unstable, it helps devalue anything they say. Instantly aiding to the maintenance of their self-perceived seat of greatness.

The outer shell the narcissist has acts as a shield to protect or hide their inner brokenness. After they use it for long enough it quite literally becomes them and they most usually won't ever turn back to choose a path of possible healing. Strangely, most people who have been diagnosed with this disorder have history of blunt trauma to the head resulting in a scar or worse. Some think this might contribute to their lack of empathy towards other living human beings. Some think it's a coincidence. They also mostly all share great trauma within their childhood and usually had a difficult family life. These true facts are usually what they use to draw in and manipulate their mostly empathetic victims.

At some point in all of our lives we all go through unfavorable situations. Whether we are self-aware of it or not, we all have the choice of how to respond to these situations. Some people argue that someone suffering from narcissistic personality disorder didn't have a choice so they create this outer layer, and that after enough time they just became stuck like that. I feel like there are so many variables that go into that opinion, that I could write an entire book and title it 'the making of a narcissist, nature vs nurture' and it would be a book that could go on for quite a while. This book won't focus as much on the educated opinion scenarios, but more on the factual sides of things. When I say factual, I mean things that have already been majorly statistically proven. The aim of this book is to hopefully bring people to a more self-aware stance on this subject, and that they will be able to choose a better path in their life.

If you ever find yourself in the aftermath of a narcissist or psychopath who turns strangers against you that never even knew your name before they learned the rumors, remember that any literate and logical person wouldn't just automatically believe bad things about someone. If you find yourself experiencing harassment from any of the people the narcissist lied about you to, you have told them not to contact you, have blocked them from the source they harass you from, and they keep finding ways to contact you with the sole purpose of harassment, don't hesitate to alert your local police department.

People need to be held accountable for harassment. It may bring peace of mind to know that if these people speak to an officer and hear out of their own mouths how ridiculous their choice of actions are, it might also help bring some clarity to them. For example, let's say the police officer asks the harasser to explain their side of the situation. This person presumably will say something similar to the fact that someone they know who claims to know you, told them things about you. The police officer will maybe ask if they have ever met you themselves. They will most likely say no. So now we have the harasser voicing to a third party the fact that they decided to blindly believe random stories about someone they never met, and then decided to harass said stranger due to those stories. How embarrassing would that be for any level headed person? Aside from embarrassing, hopefully it would be enlightening and bring to light how blinded they have become.

  Back to our villain, who eventually falls victim to themselves...One thing they also love to do is win the approval of all of your friends and family. This approval us used to distract the people closest to you, so they can pick apart your mind in private.

They are hoping and betting everyone is less smart than they are. In their minds, everyone they meet is too stupid to figure out their cunningly evil ways. In their mind, they are superior to everyone. The women in their lives serve as pawns to get what they want out of. These women will usually always think they are special compared to other women who have previously had relationships or shared a bed with these men. That's the narcissists' goal and hook tactic. They make most of the victims believe they are somehow more superior than every other ex they had ever been with. That they are needed and special to them in ways no one else had been capable of prior. They make them think that there must have been something wrong with the women that came before them. Or that the other women just didn't understand him like she does. She might even think he just likes her more than any other woman he has ever used or been with. That's where she becomes the same as every other person the narcissist uses.

In actuality some of those other women have just become wise to the situation and left. Some have known the narcissist since they were kids and have a false hope that since both of them came from toxic families, and they personally chose to overcome that and use it as an example of what not to be, instead of using it for sympathy of others or to justify poor decisions, that the narcissist can choose to make good choices then too. Those same people are led to believe no one else had helped the narcissist in a way that would make them see their inner potential. These people are usually the self-destructive helpers who will put a narcissists needs in front of their own and sacrifice themselves in hopes that the narcissist will eventually see the light of day.

Any sacrifice they make will not only never be acknowledged; they are in vain.

The narcissist is well aware of the choices they can make. They know what they're doing and consciously make decisions that hurt you. They don't care about you or anything that gets in the way of their grand scheme. If they cared about you they wouldn't do things that they know would hurt you. You are led to believe these people are smart right? Use your logic. How can a smart person not know they are doing something that will hurt you? Don't lose your logical insight due to your personal, unrequited emotions.

Another type of woman a narcissist has on hand are the side women. The women who have always been a side option, and have always been happy with that distance. This is also preferred by the narcissist. These side women not only have a vastly minimal chance to ever discover the monster they are playing servant to; they also serve as great spokespeople to aid in the manipulation of the new women that the monster brings closer to home. Or whom he chooses to live with. Once the narcissist gets these pawns in their proper places and believing what he wants them to, it's easy to get what he wants from them and others.

These men don't hold long term close relationships with other men. They often have patchy history with any man who becomes close enough to finally see what they really are. Usually this results in fights, either physical or verbal, and the end of another fake friendship. In the event they are forced to cut ties with a victim, they slander their name the same as they slander the women who leave. Male or female, the tactics are always the same. Often times the friends of narcissists only keep good standing with him due to the fact they don't also want to be slandered. They've seen the narcissist treat a friend or romantic partner as the best most perfect person alive. Sometimes for years at a time. Only to see them turn around and instantly create vicious rumors about them as if they never cared at all in the first place. They carry out this type of revenge if the victim doesn't comply with a request, disagrees with a topic the narcissist feels is offensive to their ego, or simply ends the toxic relationship.

Narcissists have been seen creating hassles and stresses within ex-friends' friend circles, jobs, the daycare the primary parent uses for their child's care, and other aspects of their life.

I firmly believe narcissists are the root cause for countless deaths and suicides yearly. Unfortunately, in most cases it would be difficult to prove, since most narcissistic victims eventually become mentally and emotionally trapped due to these people. Some victims may seek help due to the narcissistic abuse they have endured. They may be prescribed a fountain of anti-depressants and anti-anxiety medications. This method has been known to have counter effects. When patients are prescribed multiple prescriptions at once they can and have caused patients to die in their sleep. Phamaceutical companies are heavily guarded and if you wish you delve deeper in that sub context be my guest. I'll continue on with further talk of the present topic. Before I continue, I'll ask the ethical debate; who do we hold accountable for the death? The person who prescribed the plethora of pills? Or the person who was the underlying cause to the slow but deadly deterioration of an otherwise healthy persons mind which then later required the prescription? I've stated my thought on that topic. You are free to choose yours.

If you've ever found yourself in a situation where you hold back your thoughts in fear of the reaction or retaliation of the 'friend' you are considering the conversation with, ask yourself some things. How is someone who poses a threat a friend? Should you fear the reaction or repercussion of someone who claims to be your true friend? Would a real friend try to destroy you and ruin any friendships you may have if you disobey or disagree with them? Even when they are wrong? No. That's not a friendship. If you feel fear or concern about disagreeing with or ending a friendship with a person who claims to be your friend, you are most likely dealing with a narcissist. In romantic relationships especially, you will notice a change from where you once felt like you could tell this person everything you ever thought of or could think of in the world to suddenly feeling the opposite. One day, or gradually without you realizing it, you will no longer feel that sense of safety and peacefulness that you thought was once there.

When dealing with narcissists or any similar toxic partner, you will eventually feel a confined sense of entrapment over your being when considering conversations or situations where you are trained to be aware of the possible outcome. You will feel this sensation when you have a question you have wanted to ask for days. You will feel it when you want to talk about how you feel. You will begin to feel it any time you want to discuss anything pertaining to you.

You will describe it some days as if it feels like a tightness on your chest, accompanied by a dampening and or darkening of the soul. I feel the darkening is more of a shield or blanket being placed over your true self. The dampening can sometimes feel like a pressure or longing. Sometimes it shows itself as fear, anger, or resentment.

This is your inner spirit's attempt at protecting you.

The range of darkness you feel accompanying this tightness coincides with the levels of destruction being waged within you onto your soul. The tightness is not an indication of fear. In our waking lives it is the most similar feeling to compare it to. It is actually a hug to you from within yourself. It's your soul trying to stop your waking self from attempting to reason with someone who doesn't wish to be reasoned with. The feeling is stemming from your subconscious. The fear you associate this tightness with stems more from your active consciousness. By the time your episodes begin in correlation to your interest in conversation with your toxic partner, you already have experienced the negative reactions associated with the conversations you're interested in initiating. Therefore, the fear you associate with your reaction is a present tense, or actively conscious response. In conclusion, you are not scared, rather aware subconsciously that the outcome will not be good when interacting with your toxic partner. I say subconsciously, not consciously, because at the time this is happening, the victim is too engrossed in the delusion of hopeful happiness to accept their actual current reality.

Once you start acknowledging this fear sensation for what it is, it's very important to address it. This means, you have to accept that the person you want them to be isn't real. You can achieve this on your own by analyzing how many times you have had the same talks with them. How many times you have said the same things over and over. How many times you have been hurt by the same or similar situations. How many times have you heard the same apologies followed by unchanged behavior?

An apology without changed behavior is just manipulation.

There are always choices you can make to change your life or present situation. You can choose to accept the present situation for what it is and end things on your own. You can end things and seek counseling to help you healthily get past the oncoming hurdles that come with leaving a toxic partner. You can also seek counseling with your partner before you end things, although it is important to be entirely honest with your counselor or therapist in order to get the most accurate advice on your personal situation. This is their job and there is no need to be embarrassed about anything you need clarity about. You can do this. You are stronger than you let yourself believe.

We have touched base on the fact that narcissists also are compulsive liars who utilize manipulation to reach their goals. Another thing to remember is that they often times have overlapping symptoms. For instance, someone who is a narcissist may also have sociopathic traits and OCD tendencies. The same goes for the latter. Someone who is sociopathic may have overlapping narcissistic traits, OCD, or even other mood disorders. Each case is different and unique. These people are after all still human, even if they don't think they are. If they wanted to seek treatment it could help and greatly improve their symptoms. Unfortunately, most people with narcissistic disorder won't ever seek treatment. They don't think anything is wrong with them. To them, everyone else is the problem. They don't allow themselves to hurt when they lose someone they have been using and manipulating for a decade. In a lot of cases, they naturally don't feel hurt by the loss.

This is sometimes due to their lack of empathy. They will sometimes seem physically or emotionally upset due to this loss. It isn't however due to the fact they cared about this person. It's because their condition is deeply wounded. They do not take rejection well and don't ever truly admit that they are wrong let alone genuinely apologize.

They simply can't bear the thought of what others may think. They are extremely concerned with their image and what others think of them. Image is very important to these individuals. Some of my previous sentences may seem to contradict themselves, but I assure you the narcissist and sociopaths are as layered as their mountains of lies.

They need to maintain their following of loyal fans to help inflate their false sense of their grandiose self-image. At home, they will subtly threaten you then act like it was a joke. Every threat is a joke to them. They are warnings and they will scare something inside you. Listen to those feelings. You are not crazy. They will not change. Those threats are how they start to make you rethink your thoughts. It's also how they start to break down your psyche.

There are two currently identified types of narcissists. One is the aforementioned grandiose type. The other is considered vulnerable narcissism where the individual presents avoidant, defensive and hypertensive attitude towards interpersonal relations. I've witnessed far more grandiose narcissists. Or maybe I think that due to their contrasting personalities. I do stand firm that throughout every readers life there have been encounters with at the very least one person who presents each type.

Now, keep in mind not every narcissistic connection is the same. The dynamic is always the same but the details differ from scenario to scenario. So please don't pick yourself apart or compare your story to others. Although they may have different details, the overall bubble that encloses the narcissist and victim is always the same.

Narcissists are the center of their personal universe. Every person they have connection with does something for them. They get something out of every connection they make. Whether it be directly from that person or that person is the channel through which they negatively affect someone else, there is always something they believe they gain. This gives them a purpose and a reason to choose these individuals. If you have children with a narcissist and break free from their cycle, they will not flinch when inflicting pain upon the child if they think you will be hurt in the process. If you cut your child's hair, their narcissist parent will criticize the haircut just because it was you who cut it. Anything you buy them will be criticized and mocked, with complete disregard to the child's feelings, as long as the narcissist thinks he is making you look bad with the criticisms. In some cases, a narcissist will physically harm a child if the other parent makes them upset for any reason. Always believe your child, take them to the doctor, emphasize telling the truth, tell the police and document everything. Keeping our children safe, happy, healthy, and unharmed should be the main focus of a parent's life. This includes all aspects such as their mind, body and spirits. They are tiny innocent people and don't deserve anything but the best life. To a narcissist or toxic ex-partner, a child is nothing more than a pawn to try and use against you. You will be subject to grand humiliation regarding the child, false rumors, and another smear campaign to either attempt to turn everyone against you, or to ensure no one else can have or want what they have lost. It's not because he cares at all about you. You are a piece of property he has lost, or a connection who he can no longer get anything out of, and he cannot fathom the thought of someone else benefitting from his lost property. His ego cannot handle it.

Most narcissists are severely damaged within themselves. The damage and trauma are what usually give birth to the narcissistic personality disorder. They also use these events to sometimes form trauma bonds. Traumatic bonding occurs as a result of ongoing cycles of abuse in which the intermittent reinforcement of reward and punishment creates a powerful emotional bond that are resistant to change. These trauma bonds sometimes double as primary sources to be used to their benefit. These people are used as reference to support their 'good guy' backstory. With that usually comes the very amiable sob stories. The people used to verify how sad of a life the narcissist has had or who are used to justify how good of a guy the narcissist is really think they are special to the narcissist in some sort of a compassionate way. In reality the narcissist does think they're special. Just not in an emotional or empathetic sense. To them they are key components in the making of their alter ego. So, yes, they are 'special' objects to the narcissist. They are often the number one references given to new victims as a source to back up their crafted image. They are a prized possession; a resource. If the trauma bond is also female, and the narcissist male and hetero, they will most likely have had a sexual relationship of some sort. This is done as a type of the aforementioned reward system by the narcissist. These pawns are heavily tangled within a net of manipulation. The female trauma bond will offer the most to the narcissist for the longest amount of time out of all the pawns being used. They will also be given the least. This will include but not be limited to, a home to stay whenever the narcissists wants to, sex, food, money, and more. They will offer all of this thinking they are an important part of this toxic person's life. They'll pretend not to care when the narcissist keeps dating other women and doesn't ever fully commit to them. They will think they are an important longtime friend. Unfortunately, they are exactly the same as everyone else.

For the sake of authenticity, I need to include that there are some people who don't always fit every aspect of the typical victim of a narcissist. Some people just simply met their narcissist during their childhood or adolescence. These people are aware of the visible story that anyone could see from a public view. They know the narcissist has been bad to people. They even have been wronged personally in the past by this narcissist. They decide to make their own assumptions about these situations. They come to a conclusion that leaves it ok to accept this toxic relationship. They might decide the negative choices this person makes are their attempts to cry for help. These people also probably have had some personal experience with narcissistic and/or toxic family members so being around one seems familiar, and almost welcoming. A home away from home. They nestle in with their narcissist and roll with it, thinking it will all eventually be ok.

Unless your idea of a happy home is constantly hiding your true self in hopes one day you will be happy, settling for a narcissist is not a good choice. Instead of harming others like a toxic person, empaths or self-destructive partners of narcissists harm themselves. Not physically, but emotionally and mentally when they choose to engage with narcissists. These people are most usually empaths, or helpers. They also sometimes think narcissistic people just haven't been shown enough love yet. Other times they might think they just haven't ever felt real comfort or have never had a healthy environment to thrive in. These are some of the thoughts that drive these people down the path of discovering what real self-torture truly is. I say this, because more often than not, the empath chooses to stay even after being shown repetitive poor behavior by their chosen narcissist. They stay and choose the suffering because they don't know anything other than unhealthy relationships, their family were the first ones. They also truly believe it will all be worth it one day. They believe that the person hurting them doesn't know any better and that once they realize it, they will change.

They do know better. They just don't care.

The narcissist, the person with a psychopathic personality type, or someone who has traits from either one of those conditions chances of changing are the same as any other human being. They will only change if they want to. Nothing anyone does will influence them to change.

YOU CANNOT CHANGE ANYONE.

THE ONLY PERSON IN CONTROL OF CHANGING ANYONE IS THE DIRECT PERSON THEMSELVES. THIS INCLUDES TOXIC PEOPLE.

● ● ●

This is not only a reminder for those caught in the storms of abusers, this is also a reminder for the abusers themselves. If you are a narcissist, you can seek help. It won't be easy, you won't think you need help, and you will have to be HONEST once you do seek it. This choice will result in your fabricated world crumbling. Can you handle that consequence? Do you think you owe it to those around you to stop the lies and endless cycle of hurt? If you are a true narcissist or sociopath you won't care about the effects your behavior has on others. How about you do it to save the number one person in your life, yourself? Think of the weight you sometimes feel that engulfs you within. The weight that eats your soul to the point that you feel the need to try and suck the life and joy out of others. Wouldn't you like to work to abolish the raging monster within you? It starts with honesty. Once all the fake ties you created over the years hear the truth about everything they will most likely leave. Some might stay. Do you think you are strong enough to change and choose an honest path? If the people you have hurt could rise up each and every time after you did your best to destroy them, do you think you are capable of doing the same thing? Are you as strong as your victims? The only way to reconstruct yourself is to let go of what no longer suits you. Just as any other human on any other path, the core rules are the same. You must choose. You must have enough self-discipline to carry out the tasks you set for yourself.   Think of the life you could live if you just were honest about everything? If you acted in a way that you didn't have to lie and create elaborate false stories to 'prove' what you think or did is the 'right' way. Think of all the energy you could redirect into positivity, instead of hoarding excessive amounts of negative energy forcing lies and hate out of each corner within yourself. Stop recording every single conversation you have with people who have left you. There is no 'proof' in the recordings, texts, letters, and videos aside from the proof that you won't LET GO.

So let go, Mr. or Mrs. narcissist. LET GO and make room for life. Make room for positive energy, honesty, and real connections.

NO ONE CAN CHANGE YOU BUT YOURSELF. NO ONE IS IN CHARGE OF YOUR CHOICES BUT YOU.

TAKE CONTROL OF YOUR OWN LIFE.

IF YOU DON'T LIKE SOMETHING, CHANGE IT.

YOU ARE RESPONSIBLE FOR THE LIFE YOU HAVE AND THE CHOICES YOU MAKE.

STOP BLAMING EVERYONE AND EVERYTHING ELSE AND TAKE RESPONSIBILITY FOR YOUR WORDS AND ACTIONS.

● ● ●

When someone shows you toxic behavior, you need to address it promptly. Take note of how they respond. Do they turn the situation onto you instead of taking accountability for their actions or lack thereof? That's called deflecting. You are a responsible human being. You are in charge of your life. You can choose to make the decision to wait to see if they will keep disrespecting you, lying to you, not doing what they say they'll do, putting you down, ignoring your emotional needs, and telling you that *you* are why they treated you badly. Uncloud your logical lens and choose to be present. See them for what they are and act accordingly.

You can end it before the real torture begins. Some people become addicted to the praise they receive from their narcissist. When they finally give a complement after so much criticism, it makes you feel validated. It gives you hope that they can become that good version of themselves that you remember from the beginning. The image you choose to envision when things are bad. Instead of seeing reality for what it is.

On the other side of the spectrum, when they turn on you, it feels like betrayal. After all, how could someone who was so sweet and the most genuinely caring individual act in such a completely opposite manner? How could they make you fall so in love with them only to make you feel so small and unimportant? It's just what they do. Don't feel bad.

You can choose to learn to love yourself. If you do, one day when you look back you will not be able to imagine how you let them treat you like that. You may even wonder what you ever saw in them in the first place. Of course, for many of you reading this you might still be in the denial phase or you might currently be in a toxic relationship. People in the denial phase really truly still believe their narcissist is an honest person who just needs a little help. For you and those currently in a toxic relationship, I send a prayer. I pray that you find clarity, peace, happiness and understanding. Most of all I pray you find it in yourself to leave your toxic relationship behind and reclaim your life.

....

One of the things I will now focus on that narcissists, psychopathic people, or toxic people like to do is name calling. Specifically labeling a victim with a mental disorder or illness that they do not possess. When people loosely throw around a commonly heard of mental disorder with complete disregard to the actual definition of the term it irks me. It is possible the abuser is unaware of the intricacies of the term they're trying to label someone with. Though aware or not of the intricate definition of a mental disorder, the principle of the situation stays unfavorable for me.

Bipolar disorder is a term used as a crutch almost universally by most toxic people. They will quickly label their victim bipolar to try and shame their healthy, logical reaction to maltreatment. This follows how I previously mentioned narcissists love to paint their victims as mentally unstable or 'crazy'. The narcissist will save recorded phone calls, voicemails, letters they did or didn't write themselves claiming the victim wrote them, and texts for years. Even if they haven't had a close personal relationship with the alleged for over 6 years, it isn't uncommon for the narcissist to hoard these recordings. They may find themselves fixated on these items due to one or a number of their cross-referenced accompanied disorders. OCD, or obsessive-compulsive disorder, is usually the reason behind the obsession to save every interaction with any possible perceived threat. This threat is usually the ex-victim whom they are trying to mentally degrade in order to nullify all of their words. They will claim they either don't care at all about this person or they'll tell everyone they hate them. They will try their hardest to convince anyone they share the saved data with that its only purpose is to warn people of the person's invalidity. Also, of course, to 'prove' that they are crazy.

They have been saved for the purpose of ensuring no one finds out the true person behind the narcissist mask.

As far as how coincidentally all of their ex's and probably you have been labeled as bipolar, its necessary to touch on that disorder for a moment as well. I also will remind everyone that while the internet is a wonderful search engine to find things we are looking for; it isn't the place to go for a clinical diagnosis. If you think you have a disorder that impairs or negatively affects your daily life, please seek medical attention. If you would rather a more anonymous or less personal attempt to get quality analysis or discuss your personal situation, please email

lotusroomgold@gmail.com

Here you will find a reputable source with over 20 years of experience. The founder of Lotus Room has experience leading group mediations and one on one style coaching. The goal at the heart of Lotus Room really is to help people. Compassion and promoting self-growth are among the key fundamentals offered. You don't need to have an end goal or even want treatment to talk there. An example for this would be if someone is feeling depressed or suicidal and just want someone who they can talk to. The personal topics covered during conversation can include anything (apart from harassment of anyone associated with Lotus Room) and don't have to include a narcissistic component. Each experience is unique to the individual who reaches out.

Reaching out or spreading the word to anyone you know who may benefit from this annex of care will help this platform of help be more accessible to working class people. Lotus Room is a digital way to get to the root of the knot in your life that you might wish to speculate on with guidance. You are in charge of whether you would like help to simply loosen the knot, aka help visualize core components of your particular topic. Or if you would like help executing a plan to work out the knot completely until it is undone altogether. There is also another option to just have a talk session about anything at all to help ease your mind or give you someone to chat with as a means to help you find some mental clarity.

....

Back to toxically labeling people, it's very important to remind people the difference between someone reacting to an unfavorable situation and someone who actually suffers from bipolar disorder. Bipolar disorder is characterized by varying degrees of uncontrollable highs and lows. Focus on the word uncontrollable. This is not something someone who suffers from this disorder has control over. This is a very serious condition which requires a diagnosis from a licensed medical professional. To think that someone who experiences emotions other than happiness is automatically bipolar is far from logical. It's actually quite ignorant. Trying to write off someone's healthy emotional reaction to being treated badly as a sign that they are mentally unstable is unhealthy. It actually helps support the theory that the person attempting to negatively label the victims healthy reaction as unhealthy, is actually the one suffering from a mental disorder.

Bipolar disorder is defined generally as a mental condition marked by alternating periods of elation and depression. The elation periods are also called manic periods. Manic periods can last for weeks or months. The depressive episodes also last for weeks or months. So, we can conclude that someone who suffers from bipolar disorder will have severe, uncontrollable highs and lows that last a large number of days. Bipolar disorder is not characterized or defined as a person experiencing a healthy reaction to being treated poorly. Such as when you are having a normal day, then become upset due to a current situation. This information alone should bring clarity to those reading this.

The altercations in mood changes in a person suffering from bipolar disorder are usually triggered from the chemical imbalance in their brains. Sometimes they can be triggered by self-perceived good or bad situations. An example of which could be if they see a commercial or ad that sends a message in their mind which creates the shift. Where a person's mind without bipolar disorder would release a certain amount of chemicals to allow the person to feel the emotions they perceive as a reaction to the same situation, a person who suffers from this disorder will have an excessive amount of chemicals released that they may even be aware of at the time while still uncontrollable to them as it occurs. At the times that they are aware of the shift and wish desperately to make the feelings they are experiencing stop, they cannot. They are trapped underneath the emotions fighting from the other side.

Unfortunately, they are most usually incapable of pulling themselves out of these moods. This incapability has nothing to do with their personal inner strength. These individuals are exceptionally strong warriors. The lack of control is due to the chemicals in their brains. Therapy and medication can greatly improve someone who suffers from this condition. It is a serious condition and is devastating to the sufferer's personal life when untreated.

It is insulting to those who suffer from this disorder to have those who don't suffer from it be so loosely labeled with it. This condition is something that tortures their life some days. Most sufferers of bipolar disorder have difficulty maintaining friendships and jobs due to their illness. If you or someone you know may be suffering from this disorder, please reach out to a medical professional for a clinical diagnosis.

A person who reacts to a hurtful situation with upset emotions, who after a few hours or a good sleep wake refreshed and ready for a new day are simply an example of a person who does not suffer from bipolar disorder. Rather they are sufferers of a toxic partner or situation.

Narcissists try to label their victims as sufferers of bipolar disorder in an attempt to gaslight them. Also, to insinuate that their victims are getting upset for 'no reason'. A person who is having a good or otherwise neutral day who reacts to being treated badly, is not someone having a sudden and severe mood swing for no reason. They are reacting to how they are being treated. Narcissists use the labeling tactic to avoid responsibility for their actions. Blaming, deflecting, not wanting to be held accountable for their choices, and making up excuses for their behavior are a few of their favorite pastimes.

Some victims aren't aware of the in-depth definition of someone who is bipolar. They may initially know they aren't someone who suffers from that condition. After constantly being told that they are bipolar for long enough they might begin to question their own sanity, which is a result of the mental abuse from their toxic partner. The abuser is manipulating you to question your own sanity instead of actually seeing that you have every right to be upset. They do this to take the light off of their wrongdoing.

Hopefully this book can also help those on the outside looking in to be patient with their friend or acquaintance who seemed so happy from a distance, then after they left their narcissistic ex, they suddenly reveal this dark side they are finally free of. It will make you wonder "why" and "how" and "what happened so suddenly" for them to say this. After all, "they seemed so happy", "she said he was so great", "they were just fine last week", "he seemed so nice". Don't fret friends, what you're saying is in the shallow sense true. Hopefully after reading this far into the pamphlet, you can extract how these factors intertwine with the situation as a whole.

Friends, family, acquaintances, business connections and coworkers, be patient and don't judge too quickly. All of those thoughts are also exactly what the narcissist plans for you to think. They not only acted in those ways to sink the hook in their victims, it is also to fool those who think they're closest to them as well. Then if the victim ever leaves, their closest circle sees them as something to question, which backs up the stories they plan to spew if things go south. It is all just a part of their plan. The highlight reel, aka the good stuff, just isn't who they really are.

No one wants a cruel partner, which is why when it becomes a whirlwind of negativity people want to get out. Remember your friend or family member for who they are and try to see they would not agree to give their time to someone who treated them badly. So yes, in the beginning and even sometimes for years it was probably great. The mask can only stay on the narcissists face for so long until it cracks and their true self shines through. That happens far before your friend or family member leaves or asks for help. So, try to remember this when you think about how the narcissist whole initial performance is not only to become favored by you, it's to show you how they want to be perceived, so that in the event their victim leaves, their victim will look as if they are the problem instantly, without even being given the chance to explain the hellfire they left. Their smiles and fake charm are what they plan to use to win over anyone their victim knows. That way no one will question the perfect, handsome or beautiful, smiling do-gooder. They instantly question the victim, who now looks questionable.

Colleagues, family, or friends will wonder what happened and will even sometimes believe the victim is suddenly mentally unstable. Which is exactly what the narcissist wants you to think. Soon people say things like 'even their sister thinks they're insane so it must be true'. People forget that blood doesn't always equal family.

A narcissistic puzzle.

Almost 100% of all narcissists will devalue the mental stability of their victims. After all, who will believe a crazy person? Its laughable for the narcissist. Their meddling with others' lives is a game to them. A game they will try to win at all costs. Winning to them is gaining more and more blind followers to just agree and obey them. If they have children, they will do whatever they think it takes to 'win', even if it hurts their own children.

This damage they inflict on their children includes but is not limited to shaming the child for having similar traits as the other parent. They will call the child names and then claim when they act that way, they are acting like the parent who got away. This is extremely damaging to the child's psyche and actually usually creates an environment to incubate a tiny narcissistic child. The child feels bad for having similar traits as their other parent due to being scolded and shamed for it from the narcissistic parent. Even if the narcissist only trash talks the other parent in front of the child it damages the child. This other person is half of the child, so the child then feels ashamed for even being made from the other parent. The child feels confused and hurt by situations like those. These scenarios are a form of child abuse.

If one parent doesn't like or agree with the other parent that they have already separated with, they need to keep their negative comments about that parent to themselves while they're around the child they share with this person. Simply, don't talk badly about the other parent around your child. Ever. Talk however you want when the child isn't there. This is common knowledge for a healthy parent. For a narcissist, children are just a pawn to use to get back at the other parent. They can't distinguish what's appropriate to say around a child or an adult since they aren't emotionally intelligent. If they were, they would know it's inappropriate and damaging to the child to shame them, criticize them, and talk badly about the other parent around them.

Speaking of narcissists with kids, they will usually have a ridiculous number of sexual partners and will have children with multiple women. Sometimes these children are with women they want to try and manipulate with use of the children, sometimes the kids are an accident. If the mothers don't comply with whatever they request, they will try to make the mothers lives hell. They will do this at any cost, even if it hurts the child. Some will abuse the child if they are mad at the other parent for any tiny reason. Such as by placing the child's hand onto a table and striking it. If the woman breaks up with the narcissist, he will leave and ignore the child. The women they immediately turn to for sex, sources of convenience, and sometimes places to live, will be told horror stories about how the mother of his children is some form of 'batshit crazy'. He will claim this crazy ex not only will not let him see his kids, he will claim she has done 'everything in her power' to not let him see the child. That way the narcissist is free of the thing he hates most, responsibility. He can place all responsibility onto the woman whom is actually the victim, and also use her as an excuse as to why he is choosing to abandon his children. Anything a narcissist doesn't want to do or accept responsibility for; he will create an intricate lie about for his new unsuspecting victim. These lies will serve as the 'reasons' why its someone else's fault that he can't, won't, or didn't do it and why he won't accept responsibility.

Again, narcissists are compulsive liars. The lies are one reason they won't ever apologize or admit they're wrong. If they admit to one fault, they most likely will have to admit to others. They are terrified of being found out for the fraud they are. The horror they feel isn't because they are afraid to lose the people they care about. Narcissists don't care about anyone. They're afraid of losing their pawns and the people who do everything for them. If no one did the narcissists bidding, he would have to finally be held accountable for all his wrongdoings, all his lies, and all of his actions. He or she would also have to actually take responsibility and do things themselves. That is something a narcissist would never dream of doing. Being held responsible for their wrongdoings would also mean admitting to the years and years of lies they created to build themselves into the person the people who believe the lies think they are. So, they form resentment within themselves towards themselves due to the years of poor life choices they had made. This resentment is also taken out on their current and past victims. It eventually turns into hatred towards themselves as well as these people.

What a miserable cycle to choose to live in.

As a reminder, when I mentioned earlier that the narcissist is smart, it's not a compliment. Being smart isn't anything to be proud of. It's not an accomplishment on its own. It's what you do with your intelligence that matters. Although narcissists and sociopaths are considered smart mentally, they have zero emotional intelligence. They have zero empathy and they count on their mental intelligence to keep them superior to all the people they see as dumb and mentally inadequate, which is all the people they use and take advantage of. They lie to keep their pawns and pieces of property in line and doing what they want them to do. They are nothing to be celebrated, which is why intelligence is not an accomplishment alone, there needs to be contributing factors.

As another reminder, in my opinion, narcissists aren't that intelligent. If they were, they would understand that taking advantage of people for personal benefit, or to use as pawns to attempt to destroy someone else's happiness, is rather dumb.

Since they can't fathom how that would be dumb, it sadly proves my point.

One widely known saying for people who deal with or have dealt with a narcissist is that the only way to 'win' is not to play at all. Not playing means literally not speaking with them and ending all contact. Anything you say or do can and will be used against you by a narcissist. Their entire goal has shifted from what they can get from you to how they can destroy your image or happiness.

The key here is to remember that they cannot take your happiness away. You can choose to be happy. They do not control you. You are in control of your own life. You are in control of your choices, and that includes the choice to be happy.

There will be times they make you upset when it concerns your child, such as any time they hurt your child in any way. The outsiders will ask the same questions as they did when you left. Don't mind how it looks to others. You do not need to be afraid of what others might think. You know the truth. Don't feel defeated if after a stable year of almost no interaction they suddenly do something to set you off in an attempt to make you 'look crazy' again. He does this in hopes to make others whom you might see daily or on a consistent basis question who you are as a person.

You have to remember that you're human. You have emotions. Emotions range from happy to sad to angry and all points in between. Its ok and healthy to feel emotions other than happy once in a while. It's not ok to use your emotions as an excuse to act out and hurt others. Feeling these other emotions sometimes and as a reaction to how someone is treating you is OK. You are not crazy. What matters is how you respond to the reactions that you feel. Thinking and feeling are one thing (well two), but choosing to act on your feelings and thoughts is another.

Take a deep breath and think before you act. As a parent of a child shared with a narcissistic abuser, the mental abuse often doesn't leave when the relationship ends. They will even go as far as to attempt to take away familiar places their child enjoys and might have enjoyed for years, just to attempt to sever a healthy tie the other parent may have with someone or something that isn't them.

The narcissist or sociopath wants you to feel as alone as they feel inside.

No matter how significant or insignificant the tie might be to you, if it is healthy, the narcissist doesn't want you to have it. He will sacrifice his child's own happiness by attempting to remove this familiar place from their child, if it means he will 'win' and remove a healthy connection you have. Children are innocent and should be kept from harm. Not put in harm's way and disregarded as a piece of property.

An example of an attempt to fray a connection you have and take away a safe space from the child would be to not secure a time with you to pick up the child you share from a daycare. Then purposely pick the child up at a time that wasn't secured with you, lie to the daycare staff who allowed the pick up without notifying you, and tell the staff he'll contact you but never does.

Whew. Most people who don't think before they act would scream at the daycare staff for allowing the pick up without hearing from you, the primary parent, first. They might even tell the staff that the daycare isn't needed any more and sever the tie.

Though if this was done, the parent would be doing exactly what the narcissist planned for them to do. It wouldn't do anything but hurt the child and remove another longstanding healthy connection.

If thinking before we act was put into play here, the parent who is under mental attack from the narcissist can choose to remain calm with the daycare staff and keep the connection for the child. The parent can remain calm when approaching the situation with the narcissist and remind them of their personal agreement regarding their personal shared placement agreement with the courts. Usually there is a very general court order applied to most cases that there needs to be an agreed upon time and a direct response from the primary parent before the secondary can pick the child up. Common sense and decency is all that's required for that process to run smoothly.

If we think before we act when dealing with a narcissist we can avoid falling into their traps and also make sure our children don't get hurt by the narcissist's schemes.

The narcissist bets on manipulating any and everyone, especially those closest to you. He orchestrates that whole scenario to attempt to make you look more untrustworthy and mentally unstable. He wants you to suffer for leaving him. Even if he fails at making you mad at the person close to you, he will still feel he succeeded if he made the target more unsure about your mental stability. It's all a game to the narcissist. In doing this the narcissist still feels good about his choices and self-perceived progress.

This is just one scenario and it may seem confusing to some, yet completely relatable to others. If it is confusing to you, I'd be willing to bet you haven't had a close interpersonal relationship with a narcissist or sociopath whom you've shared a child or children with. If this scenario is relatable for you, I'm hoping this book gives you peace of mind that you are not alone, you are not insane, and reminds you that you should not give up on yourself.

Don't let the anger he provokes fuel the choices you make. When you feel anger for any situation, it is best to wait until the feeling is gone, or redirect yourself out of the anger in a healthy way, before you react.

Neuroscientists have discovered that every time you resist acting on your anger you actually rewire your brain.

It is important to re-program your brain from time to time in order to become more balanced. Anyone can rewire their brain and in doing so change their own brains functioning. This affects how you feel, and how you respond to your feelings. This can really change your life in a positive way. When you realize you have the power to control how you react to how you feel, you gain self-empowerment. It's an amazing thing to learn and build off of. This will help you with the self-control that you may have felt that you lost after years or months of narcissistic abuse. Remember that anything that has been lost can be found. It may not be how you remembered it, it may look completely different, it may be a completely new version. It is still gaining back what you lost.

All of these versions of a healthy recovery are wonderful and promising for your inner health and happiness. You are probably used to being subjected to immense criticism, ridicule and even threats, as per your narcissistic abuser. Please remember to try not to self-criticize too much. Try to embrace your true self and love it. Everything takes time and no two paths are on the same timeline. Never compare your progress with someone else's. Their story is not yours, so their progression isn't relevant to compare with yours. Each individual story is different and unique.

As you may recall when you look back, the criticism from your past abuser seemed to be more like forced recommendations or commands, and if you questioned it, they would say they were just trying to help. For example, your favorite shirt. They know it's your favorite. They might even have called you pretty one day when you wore it. Then one day as you feel like you've become cozier, he will point at that same favorite shirt of yours and tell you not to wear it ever again. Not only that, he will tell you not to wear any shirt like it ever again. You might have asked why and he will maybe tell you it's ugly, or looks bad on you. You'll feel bad and maybe confused but you won't tell him that. You're already probably living together at this point so you trust him to tell the truth. You just agree and move on. It's like this when they slowly let their controlling behavior start to engulf you.

When you are recovering and making progress, remember to try not to minimize or criticize your personal outcomes. This is important as you progress through this journey of self-rediscovery and recovery. If you catch yourself thinking a thought that sounds like a forced recommendation or command, try to redirect to a more positive viewpoint. Don't beat yourself up if you think you sound negative or harsh on yourself. Be proud that you can acknowledge that you might be sounding like that. If you can witness yourself going through the process I just stated, that in itself is actually a step inside the recovery space in your mind that you can be proud of. You can go further and top off that progress of recognizing your possibly self-sabotaging comment, and redirect yourself with a positive affirmation on top of the realization in itself. Remember, progress is progress. A journey of a thousand steps begins with one. Don't doubt yourself, you can recover. Just be patient and trust your journey.

The farther you make it away from the trauma and the closer you get to recovering, the more clearly you will see the signs you wrote off in the beginning as things began to turn for the worst.

Some scenarios could begin shortly after you had signed the lease to your apartment or home with an ex narcissistic partner. You could have been happily enjoying the few fresh new weeks of sharing the same roof, and unsuspectingly are issued a threat as you pull into the driveway to park. It can be a simple sentence masked with a smile, but the tone of voice and vibe will not be friendly. He may say something simple. For example, "Don't fuck me over, you'll regret it and it won't end pretty for you". He may stare at you unflinching until you reply or give some answer to him. You might be taken off guard and when you realize he is awaiting a response you might just shrug and say ok. After which you will have noticed he snapped out of the unfriendly vibe and immediately got out of the car or changed the subject. You may sit in the car for a moment due to being caught off guard. If you later asked him why he said that he probably just shrugged casually and smiled, brushing it off as a joke. Right?

If this sounds similar, you have absolutely been threatened by a toxic partner. With narcissists its less about the direct threat and more about the warning behind it. They choose their words carefully so as to write it off as nothing if it gets brought up to other people. This threat is one they do try to follow through with if you ever catch on to their toxicity or leave them. You may be baffled due to the length of time you thought you knew this person before these scenarios start to enfold. Maybe you knew them for a decade. None of those things are significant when entering the narcissists nest. You only knew what he showed you.

You also probably figured he knew you weren't the type of person to ever intentionally do someone wrong. Which further confuses you about why he would say something like that to you. He did know that about you, what he meant with the threat is that if you become wise to his schemes or eventually left him, he will try to make your life miserable. Like he said, it wouldn't be pretty for you. He would view you breaking up with him as an extreme personal hit, since narcissists actually have a fragile sense of self. So, even though he was direct with his threat it was still a game or riddle. Everything is a game to them. They also threaten you to do things and use the thing they threatened you to do against you. They use the situations to prove to others that you're mentally unstable. For instance, naming your child. You may have originally named your child a name your ex-narcissist didn't like. He might then threaten you regarding the name. He will say that if you didn't change your child's name, that he would give up his parental rights. This is not only legally improbable but also outrageous. Although, dealing with the mental abuse for so long from these monsters, logistics seem to lose strength, since you have seen illogical situations play out under the toxic partners games. In a logical world, the games he played never should have worked out. Yet they almost always did. Although the threat didn't seem logical, it seemed possible, right? So, you changed your child's name. Your abuser even let you choose the new name yourself, right? Another pawn in the chess game. Don't feel bad for changing your child's name, or following through on a threat where you thought you were doing what was best for your child. You didn't do it for the monster, you did it to try and protect your child. All you or anyone can do is learn, grow, and move on.

This brings me to the conclusion of the name change example. You will find your ex-narcissist now uses the fact that you changed your child's name against you. They will say it is vital reasoning when they tell their new victims as to proof of how you are crazy. He will omit his part in the equation of the name change. The new victims won't know he threatened you to change it. They will just hear what he wants them to. And as he predicts about his new victims, they are too mindless to inquire about the whole story.

What was one of the reasons the narcissist made the threat about the name change? He wanted a sense of power and control.

No one has control over yourself but you. Be conscious of your actions and choices. You cannot change the past but anyone can learn from the past and choose a new path at any time.

You would wonder how narcissists have all the energy for this negativity but they usually suck all their energy out of all of their victims. They get a grand sense of accomplishment when the feeling of superiority washes over them as they use and use more and more people. Most of the time they don't feel any empathy. That emotional void actually fuels their ability to be more and more intricate with their insanity. After all, people with empathy don't look at other human beings as pawns in the first place. It takes emotional energy and intelligence to be able to care about the effect one's choices have on other people. It's also needed to be able to see and understand how those involved will be affected by the choices we make. Doing this analytic phase when making decisions seems second nature to most readers. Unfortunately, narcissists aren't smart enough to comprehend the emotional benefit of caring for others without expecting anything in return. They don't see how they actually can gain much more in life if they were empathetic and considerate of others.

As another reminder, the people that normally latch onto these narcissistically driven people are often times people who have the 'helper' personality type. A person with a helper type personality could have all or some of these traits. The helper can be described as a person who is seen as a selfless mentor figure, always ready to lend a helping hand. Sometimes they actively search for ways to improve the lives of others. They can be generous, altruistic, and empathetic. They are hardworking and motivated people with a drive to connect with the world. They love attending to other people and feeling helpful. Sometimes also referred to as the giver.

As you can see, this person is almost completely opposite in terms of personality traits compared with a person with narcissistic tendencies. It's all making so much more sense now isn't it. The helper is attracted to the horror, the sob stories, or the altogether misfortune that surrounds this charismatic, wide smiling narcissist. They feel that this charming individual has just had hard times and is too smart and wonderful to be a bad person. Bad things must just unfortunately happen to them, right? Then these helpers think they just need a little guidance and real true love. Since the narcissist has just never experienced a healthy relationship, right? Especially since all of his stories about his ex includes how they are extremely crazy followed by lists of outrageous supporting facts to intrigue the helper into believing these lies and ultimately sucking them in to being the next victim.

As with all things, there is always an exception to every rule. As I stated earlier, the details are always different but the bubble containing the narcissist and helper are always the same. Some unhealthy connections with an ex-narcissist evolve due to meeting as kids through common friends. You may have chosen to think that since you had both came from bad family situations that he could be like you and choose to make choices that don't harm others.

That in itself is your unhealthy reason to keep giving this person chances. Regardless of if you never gave him money, even when he went to jail. If you didn't let him use your car when he had a suspended driver's license because if he would get pulled over by the police while driving your car without a license, you would get a fine. You decided you weren't going to let him bring you down with him. You told him if he paid off his fines and got his driver's license back, he could then use your vehicle. That made him angry and he probably told you that if you don't let him use your car before he gets his license back that you were a bad girlfriend and just didn't care about him. He was showing you right there that he didn't care if you were to get a fine, he just wanted you to give him what he wanted from you. When you didn't, and for logical reasons at that, he tried to manipulate you into thinking you were the bad guy. In reality, someone who doesn't care if they cause you harm, even if that harm is a possible fine in your name, he is the bad guy. Nothing you do will be enough for him.

The secret is, nothing you ever do is going to be enough for a narcissist.

Make sure you make healthy choices with everything you do.

If someone is upset or mad at you for looking out for yourself, they don't care about you. If they are upset that you're encouraging them to make better choices, that is a red flag that they are a toxic individual.

A toxic person will become enraged and try to manipulate you into feeling bad and doing what he wanted.

He will tell you that you aren't a good girlfriend and that you don't care about him if you don't disregard your own life and just do whatever he wanted.

This is typical narcissistic or sociopathic, toxic behavior.

They want you to give them everything they ask for at any and all cost to you. No matter what negative expense or effect it might have on you. Your response should be that if they don't want to be in the position they are in, they should make different choices. They need to stop blaming everyone else for their choices. If they don't want to make different choices, they don't have the right to complain about their issues. After all, we are the only ones in control of our choices. No one can make us do anything. We have to choose to give them that power.

In the end it isn't them who is powerful, it's the person who decided to give them authority over their choices.

I challenge each and every one of you to make the decision to give yourself the power over your choices. If someone demands something from you that you know might have negative possible outcomes, you have the choice and the power to say no. Anyone who cares about you won't ever question a decision you make to ensure you stay in a healthy path in life. A healthy person who cares about you won't try and manipulate you into feeling bad for not giving them something. Remember that.

If you try to stay in a relationship with a toxic partner or narcissist after they discover you won't let them use you at your own expense, it's usually all downhill from that. They realize the reality of the situation and feel threatened that you might reveal who they really are to people. That's when the narcissist will begin with the blackmail and threats. If they have already been threatening and blackmailing you, it will get much worse.

Part 2

I want to begin to transition to the second half of the book. There is more to comment on the narcissist, but as the title states, this book is also about the helper. Let's take a moment and look at the helpers and givers who have at one time loved these people. The people who might still love one of them but chose to break from the cycle to pursue a healthier life. Also, for those who are somehow still connected to their narcissist legally, due to children, or intimately.

After these reminders, the second part of the book will describe a number of healthy ways to cope with your life after or during the mental abuse from a toxic or narcissistic person. A toxic person that you once gave part, or all, of yourself to.

If you have no children with this toxic person, please remove yourself completely from their lives. Or, remove them completely from your life. However you want to envision it this is extremely important. You need to remember that the fact you love them isn't enough to stay with them. You need your love reciprocated by someone who actually loves you back. Leaving doesn't mean you never loved them or that you gave up. Leaving is showing you understand the situation enough to know you aren't with a healthy person. You see you are not receiving a healthy proportion of love from this person. You accept that this person isn't who you thought they were. You accept that you need to address the reality of the situation, not come to a conclusion or solution due to where you want to be or what you envision might happen. You reached the point where you know you will be happier and emotionally healthier elsewhere.

This is a huge step and needs to be final and executed with firm action. No matter how much you miss them you must not contact them. They know you and know how to manipulate the outcome they want from a conversation or encounter with you. They will promise you the world in exchange for your compliance. They might even bring proof as to how they have changed or will change. It is all a hoax. If you accept, it might even seem better for a while. The return honeymoon phase doesn't last. They return to the same toxic self whom they hide beneath their mask soon enough and the cycle then begins again. Hence why it is imperative to your emotional and mental health to cut the ties completely when you leave. No phone calls, texts, emails, meetings, nothing. Love yourself more than the idea you have in your mind of what you wish this person will turn into, or become again. Look at the current situation. Be present. Don't make a decision based on what you hope or want to happen.

Make a decision based on what is currently happening in your life and what actually happened.

No matter where you are on your personal current stage of recovery, I recommend that you reach out and try a healthy form of therapy. Any healthy activity to help ensure your general mental and emotional health is nurtured, won't hurt to try.

Let me add that you don't need to be suffering from a connection with an unhealthy person to try any of these activities. They are good for any and everyone.

I would like to highlight some key forms of abuse. These are often the types of abuse the abuser will really use against you, since they are oftentimes the most explained as reasonable by the abuser. They are not reasonable, you don't deserve this, nothing you did warrants this behavior from them.

Some of the types of emotional and mental abuse are:

- **Verbal abuse:** yelling at you, insulting you or swearing at you.
- **Rejection:** Constantly rejecting your thoughts, ideas and opinions.
- **Gaslighting:** making you doubt your own feelings and thoughts, and even your sanity, by manipulating the truth.
- **Put-downs:** calling you names or telling you that you're stupid, publicly embarrassing you, blaming you for everything. Public humiliation is also a form of social abuse.

- **Causing fear:** making you feel afraid, intimidated or threatened.
- **Isolation:** limiting your freedom of movement, stopping you from contacting other people (such as friends or family). It may also include stopping you from doing the things you normally do – social activities, sports, school or work. Isolating someone overlaps with social abuse.
- **Financial abuse:** controlling or withholding your money, preventing you from working or studying, stealing from you. Financial abuse is another form of domestic violence.
- **Bullying and intimidation:** purposely and repeatedly saying or doing things that are intended to hurt you.

Emotional abuse can cause anxiety, guilt, shame, fear and depression. It can damage your self-esteem, sense of safety and your general outlook on trust. One main component missing in all of these scenarios is lack of fear. This might be considered the basis of all the other stemming ailments. With the presence of unhealthy fear, a person's entire sense of self can be ultimately engulfed by shadows of negativity. So much so that they can forget who they are and become a shrouded version of what they once were.

Along with the presence of unhealthy fear is usually a lack of a healthy amount of self-trust. This lack of self-trust usually results in a lack of inner peace. This often happens as a result of the negative feelings spreading and overpowering any healthy feelings. Refer back to the pie chart example as it can be used to help visualize this experience.

The visual of the pie graph will allow a sense of greater understanding of the ripple effect caused by our present lingering emotions. The pie graph allows us to immensely simplify the range of human complexity and emotion so that we can put it into a picture. A pie graph is a representation of quantitative information by means of a circle divided into sections.

Imagine the pie graph is divided into equally distributed healthy human emotions. The graph has an unhealthy slice that gradually turns all the slices on either side of it into part of itself. Just like if you add food coloring to water, the water slowly changes from clear to the color of the die you chose to drop into it. The slices of the graph slowly change like this until there is just a sliver of original emotion left. This would be the visual of fear tainting and engulfing the healthy range of emotions any individual has.

We could go deeper into the analogy and also explain that each range of emotion could also have its own new characteristic after mixing with the fear portion. This could also go on to explain how each individual can show different symptoms from the same underlying cause, since it is impossible to duplicate the human condition. As in, each person is their own individual self so they will produce their own individual results.

As I previously mentioned, one main component that is missing from the graph is a healthy sense of self trust or inner peace. This is one of the base components affected that also greatly impacts all other ranges of emotions and reactions.

It has been said that it might be most commonly taught or viewed upon by most societies around the globe that someone who has otherwise no seemingly troubling issues in their lives are superior to those who have. It has also been said that those same individuals with no stories of conflict in their lives have better insight than those who have had troubles in their lives. The people without the traumatic or messy drama stories are looked upon as if they must know what they're talking about when asked for advice. This information is based upon a thought that since they haven't suffered as others have, all the aforementioned can be concluded.

In my educated opinion, I believe there will be found more wisdom from an individual who has weathered many disastrous storms, and their psychological or emotional result is a still, calm and loving demeanor. This is not to say that if that same person ever is seen feeling frustrated that they must not have learned from the past. Frustration alone is not an automatic indication of downfall. When felt healthily it is not a reason to use caution around someone. For if they have seen the darkness and how easy it is to succumb to it or become it and they still choose light, they are most definitely someone who has the strength inside them that's only found with the wisdom that comes with making healthy decisions.

That is my personal view on this corrupted societal norm. Although, when psychology was being reinvented by some wealthy scholars who wanted to make a business out of it, they ran some experiments with the people in their social class. They discovered that the wealthy class had the exact same mental disorders or ailments as the poor class. This didn't serve their business agenda very well, for if the poor classes found out that with proper healthcare, hygiene, and schooling, they would be indistinguishable from the otherwise perceived as superior upper class, it wouldn't financially benefit the upper class at all. This led to the breakdown of social classes and some of the lies they feed the population to this day, to people who have forgotten that it was other people not different from themselves who refined and molded the theories and lessons learned in the books. Some psychological lessons and theories are obviously very helpful and well-studied before they are used. However, that doesn't mean everything you read in a college textbook is concrete fact.

Back to my previous point, how the textbook definition of the divided socioeconomic class portion of psychology originated. The scholars involved decided to fool the general public with the lies they still teach today. They decided to lie to benefit from the economic outcome of the falsely perceived superiority of the upper class. This lie has become a burden for most of the population. Fueling parents to force their artist or mechanically inclined children into giving up their dreams and happiness to become doctors or dentists. This scenario results in doctors who hate their jobs, diagnose poorly and probably graduated at the bottom of their class. They didn't graduate at the bottom due to lack of intelligence. They did so due to lack of interest or passion. This causes the ripple effect where the general population are now cared for less than appropriately and even treated rudely at times. This fault doesn't only lie in the family aspect but also in the person who decided a life of pleasing others at the expense of themselves. This is also a form of emotional abuse from others as well as self-destructive behavior when done to oneself. There are countless scenarios within each socioeconomic class where the cause and effect reach each class. This isn't a coincidence. We are all connected whether we want to acknowledge it or not. We are all equal and in being so we all deserve to live what we feel are happy, healthy, fulfilling lives. No matter how much or how little one makes, the amount doesn't define their inner being. The example of the doctor I just used can be used to support that expression. Everyone knows doctors make a very comfortable salary. So, the fact that the doctor was miserable inside wasn't due to lack of funds. It was due to lack of fulfilment from not doing what called out to their soul.

One of my base rules in life is to remember there is always an exception to a rule. Devils' advocates will like to try and use the one exception to devalue the authenticity of a statement or finding. When they do and when appropriate remind them of the aforementioned rule. Try not to confuse an educated, inquiring mind too hastily with the devil's advocate label. Whereas its healthy to ask questions when you are truly curios, it is quite different and separate from the devil's advocate who just wants to challenge everything anyone claims. I bring this up because there are obviously people who choose a profession they are more obligated to than fond of and lead perfectly happy lives.

Keep all of this in mind when you feel as though you need advice, help, or other opinions. Remember that a psychologist, therapist, counselor or other talk therapist are still just people after all. They have their own life and own personal issues. Some therapists are also diagnosed with mental and emotional issues such as ADD (attention deficit disorder) or ADHD (attention deficit hyperactivity disorder). They are taught not to tell patients about their personal life so as to keep the illusion of being someone who has their life together. This aids in the façade that therapists of all kinds deserve the insane hourly rates patients agree to so that they can hopefully find help or peace of mind.

You're just rolling the dice and gambling with your mental health when seeing any licensed therapist. When it comes down to your diagnosis or the advice they give you, it's still just a collective result of their own personal beliefs wrapped in pretty papers that they label as superior. Of course, due to their education, they are a professional. Also due to the diploma they received, they are allowed to ask for such a high rate from those in need.

It's an expensive opinion from a person with their own mental problems and family issues.

Take that into account when they tell you how they think you should live your life. Some therapists are humble and try to be unbiased in their approach. Of course, some may argue it is impossible for any human alive to ever make a decision that is not based in some part from a personal bias they have.

Therapists aren't all bad people. Some actually care what you are thinking and genuinely want to help you. Just don't automatically listen to their opinion without thinking for yourself first. Just like when you see a doctor who practices medicine, when the matter is serious, it is good to get at least one other opinion.

I have met in my past years working in healthcare numerous people who were diagnosed by their doctor with months to live. Some sought opinions from other doctors which lead to being given a treatment that led to a cure from others. Imagine what might have happened if they had accepted the death sentence from the first doctor they saw without seeking a second opinion?

We must remember that all humans are prone to error, no matter how smart they are. Take diagnoses into careful consideration but always get a second opinion. Heck, get three or four if that's what you feel is necessary. It is your life. You are in control of what you choose to do or not do.

Remember with psychiatric care, the origin of the brainwashing of the general population into thinking if someone has gone through toxic scenarios that they will never give adequate advice, is a business tactic to keep their offices bringing in the big bucks. They try to claim that individuals who have gone through toxic situations are defected to lure you into being a paying patient of theirs. Patient doctor relationships are to be kept one sided because if you learned that your therapist, psychologist, or psychiatrist has also had turbulent negative situations in their own lives, their manipulation into making you believe someone whose life has had problems doesn't have the capacity to give adequate advice would be proven inaccurate.

Now keep in mind there is a lot of gray area. Do research and don't just automatically believe any and everything someone says to you. I'm not devaluing all therapists. I'm trying to bring light to the games the founders of the psychology field play on their students and patients. I'm also not saying you should go and find any random individual who has gone through hardships and automatically believe anything they say since they've been through it. Use your intuition, find credible sources. Assess this person's level of inner peace, honesty, and whether or not they choose love over hate regularly.

If someone is currently still in an ongoing toxic cycle, they are someone who's advice may not be as helpful as someone who has exited a toxic cycle. Someone who has ended toxic cycles and has also found a new healthy alternative life to live might give some great advice. Usually someone with those characteristics has been on a road to healing for a while or long enough for themselves personally to probably give you some good insight.

Remember that someone's advice can be taken into account but it is your choice and yours alone what you do with your life. If you choose to do something someone tells you to do and it doesn't go as planned you need to remember to take responsibility for your own choices and actions. It is ok if you are frustrated about the advice you were given and also to be a little upset with yourself for taking the advice. Just make sure you don't linger there. Take the situation as a learning experience and move forward. Wherever you are in your life currently is a direct result of your choices. If you find unhealthy connections tied to those choices it would be best to distance yourself from those ties. This can help strengthen your inner self and help you make choices that are better for you and those around you.

Taking responsibility for your own actions and choices is a great point to always work on. If you are considering doing something that you would have to hide from others, yourself, or the law, it is absolutely something you should not do. Some things from the past that we are at fault for are easier than others to admit to ourselves while going through the healing process. The more difficult situations to admit to yourself usually unlock greater healing results for your future self.

It's great when you strive to live honestly and directly daily. On top of this, when you are honest and know you won't need to lie if asked about something, the stress fueled by fear will disappear. That might be the only fuel you need to help yourself make better choices. Doing this will result in removing fear from the equation when thinking about having to be held responsible or accountable for your actions. If you always choose to do things that you have no problem accepting accountability for, you choose to live free of fear. In turn you are taking control of your life and living with positive healthy power.

Meditation

Meditation is an ancient practice that is believed to have originated in India many thousands of years ago. Throughout history it has been practiced by many neighboring countries and has integrated into many religions. Buddhist meditation is a type of meditation in Buddhism. According to Wikipedia, the closest words for meditation in the classical languages of Buddhism are bhavana (mental development) and jhana/dhyana (mental training resulting in a calm and luminous mind). Pretty neat, right? Nothing short of amazing. As with all things, there are variations of Buddhism. There are Chinese, Japanese, and Tibetan forms, which have their own focuses. If you are not only looking for a way to heal and redirect in a healthy way, but also are interested in an ancient complex school of thought, there is a magnificent amount of diverse learning materials and teachings involving the forms of Buddhism.

Here is a short list of meditations labeled in a westernized fashion that are said to aid in stress relief:

- mindfulness meditation
- spiritual meditation
- focused meditation
- movement meditation
- mantra meditation
- transcendental meditation
- progressive relaxation
- loving-kindness meditation
- visualization meditation

Each of these can be used to focus on a desired area per each individual need or desire.

For example, let's say you choose mindfulness. When you practice and learn what mindfulness is, you can use this to become more cognizant of your bodily sensations, thoughts and feelings. Meditation can help people overcome uncomfortable and sometimes intrusive thoughts or memories and help them pass without judgement. A large majority of domestic abuse survivors often suffer from PTSD (post-traumatic stress disorder) symptoms, or the disorder itself. Meditation is said to help those diagnosed with that disorder as well. One study showed that a group of veterans who participated in a weekly guided meditation class for one month were found to have decreased amounts of cortisol. Cortisol is the stress hormone. Guided meditation is led by a trained professional. I would add links for specific guided meditation locations, but due to location and time differences, and also possibly the time lapsed from the pamphlets publish date and the date you read this, doing so may cause errors or discrepancies in the references. Instead, I will simply recommend that you use the search engine that your province provides or is available to you. Type in a general word search similar to "guided meditation near me" and make sure the link you choose doesn't include the word 'AD' near the end. After you find a location or group interesting enough for your liking, make sure you check some reviews as well. Be sure to remember that if you choose one location and it doesn't feel one hundred percent right for you, simply try another location. Don't give up and remember that no two studios are the same. Just like how you can go to three different hair salons and have three different experiences. If guided meditation is what you're after, I'm sure that there is a location that will feel right for you.

Qigong

Qigong can be classified as a form of meditation. It is a Chinese system of physical exercises and breathing control related to tai chi. Tai Chi is a Chinese martial art and system of calisthenics, consisting of sequences of very slow and controlled movements. In Chinese philosophy, Tai Chi is the ultimate source and limit of reality, from which yin, yang and all of creation originate. Now before you feel intimidated, remember that simply by existing you are already a part of all celestial matter. Pretty amazing! With Qigong, as you meditate through concentrating on movements and breathing, it doesn't seem like you are meditating at all. That aspect is very favorable for those who feel that they don't know how to meditate in the first place. This is a highly recommended form of clearing your mind while also reducing stress and boosting your vitality. There are many videos available for free on the internet. Just be sure to do a little research and find authentic forms as well as a level that is comfortable for you. There are many different styles, variations of the same movement, and levels of practice.

I highly recommend beginning with a set of movements often referred to as the eight pieces of silk, eight section brocade, eight silken movements, or eight silk weaving. Some think the name of the form generally refers to how the eight individual movements of the form characterize and impart a silken quality to the body and its energy. Similar to that of a brocade, which is a rich fabric woven with a raised pattern with either gold or silk.

Here is a list of the eight, with two variations of each:

•Two hands upholding the sky, **Two Hands Hold up the Heavens (Shuang Shou Tuo Tian)**

This move is said to stimulate the "Triple Burner" aka "Triple Warmer" or "Triple Heater" meridian (Sanjiao). It consists of an upward movement of the hands, which are loosely joined and travel up the center of the body.

• Pulling the bow, **Drawing the Bow to Shoot the Eagle / Hawk / Vulture**

While in a lower horse stance, the practitioner imitates the action of drawing a bow to either side. It is said to exercise the waist area, focusing on the kidneys and spleen.

•Crane spreading its wing, **Separate Heaven and Earth**

This resembles a version of the first piece with the hands pressing in opposite directions, one up and one down. A smooth motion in which the hands switch positions is the main action, and it is said to especially stimulate the stomach.

•Looking backward, **Wise Owl Gazes Backwards or Look Back**

This is a stretch of the neck to the left and the right in an alternating fashion.

•Left and right swing, **Sway the Head and Shake the Tail**

This is said to regulate the function of the heart and lungs. Its primary aim is to remove excess heat (or fire) (xin huo) from the heart. *Xin huo* is also associated with heart fire in traditional Chinese medicine. In performing this piece, the practitioner squats in a low horse stance, places the hands on thighs with the elbows facing out and twists to glance backwards on each side.

- Up and down stretch, **Two Hands Hold the Feet to Strengthen the Kidneys and Waist**

This involves a stretch upwards followed by a forward bend and a holding of the toes.

- Diagonal knock, **Clench the Fists and Glare Fiercely (or Angrily)**

This resembles the second piece, and is largely a punching movement either to the sides or forward while in horse stance. This, which is the most external of the pieces, is aimed at increasing general vitality and muscular strength.

- Toe and heel bounce, **Bouncing on the Toes**

This is a push upward from the toes with a small rocking motion on landing. The gentle shaking vibrations of this piece is said to "smooth out" the qi after practice of the preceding seven pieces or, in some systems, this is more specifically to follow Sway the Head and Shake the Tail.

I have found that Qigong is highly favored due to its effectiveness and seemingly effortless practice. The art of practicing breathing paired with movements is enough in itself to help clear the mind and calm the spirit. This is great for those who are not into highly strenuous workouts and for those who need to work out more than just their physical bodies. This really is a healing art. In a world that never slows down, finding even twenty minutes or so a day to incorporate regulating your energy is well worth it and very rewarding. There are levels to this practice, so make sure you are practicing at a level you are comfortable with, and go from there.

Yoga

Yoga is well known around the globe. There are various types and levels to yoga. Here is a list of eight yoga poses that are suggested to help ease your mind. The internet and physical libraries or personal yoga teachers can help you discover the combination that is best for you.

- Child's Pose (Balasana)
- Thunderbolt Pose (Vajrasana)
- Easy Pose (Sukhasana)
- Seated Forward Bend Pose (Paschimottanasana)
- Wide-Legged Straddle Pose (Upavistha Konasana)
- Legs Up the Wall Pose (Viparita Karani)
- Puppy Pose (Anahatasana)

- Tree Pose (Vrksasana)

Physical Exercise

It has been proven that humans benefit mentally and emotionally from physical exercise. A few synonyms of exercise are work, movement, exertion and effort. Use the word that feels more comfortable for you. As a bare minimum to base your health journey on, remember that humans are not nocturnal and need natural sunlight, fresh fruits and vegetables, water, and MOVEMENT.

If you set a goal of one day per month that you choose one activity for, and exert energy doing it for at least 20 minutes, that still counts. You can add days or times as you feel more confident and comfortable. Some people like weekly or bi-weekly sessions. Some people enjoy exercising every other day or every couple of days. Some people prefer or need the structure of a schedule so that they don't put it off forever.

Don't stress or put yourself down. You can do this! You can compare this to a household chore like doing the dishes. You may not always want to wash them, but when you are done you feel much better. Wash the dishes in your mind by choosing your favorites off this list. ☺

Of course, yoga, qigong, and meditation are exercises that you can choose from. There are also:

•Walking   •Swimming   •Running   •Jogging •skipping rope

•Hiking   •Rafting   •canoeing   •boating •paddle boating

•lifting weights   •weight training   •boxing •kick-boxing

•ballet   •gymnastics   •basketball   •football •baseball

•volleyball   •disc golf   •sightseeing   •jump rope

•skateboarding   •bicycling   •foot scooter •swings

These are a few examples of how to be active. You do not need to be an expert to participate in any activity of any kind. You just need to enjoy it and practice it safely.

<u>*Art*</u>

Another form of decompression can be found with various forms of art. You don't need to possess a magnificent skill at any type of art to perform it or participate in it.

Art is meant to be performed not perfected. Every masterpiece has a flaw. Some might say that any form of exercise is a form of art. Which would include some of the items listed under exercises. Other forms include:

- Drawing
- Painting
- Singing
- Dancing
- Musical Instruments
- Reading
- Writing
- Poetry
- Culinary Arts
- Sewing
- Crocheting
- Knitting
- Quilting
- Pottery

Socializing and Solitude

Everyone needs a balanced combination of socialization and solitude. Whether socialization recharges you or solitude does, recharging your inner battery is necessary to fully function adequately. One needs to also decompress and let off excess energy from time to time. Everyone has their own personal formula to carry out these tasks. It is important to connect with people who respect you and will not take it personal if you need your space. It is equally important to socialize with people who won't try to force their idea of fun onto you. Hang with people who like the things you like. Or if they like different things, people who are able to respect your boundaries while doing so.

It is never too late to try something new unless you are buried six feet in the earth.

Epilogue

There are portions of this book that repeat previously stated ideas. The repeated information was done on purpose to hopefully help it stick better to the reader's mind.

By no means were all aspects of people who exhibit toxic, narcissistic, or sociopathic behaviors covered.

As can be said that not every healthy outlet in existence was named.

This book does not have all of the answers.

I am hoping this book has brought with it some peace of mind.

I hope it brings comfort,

acts as a portal revealing a hidden door for the
readers who need one,

as a light in someone's dark room,

Or

for others...

As the curtains that are drawn to let in the
sunlight.